REVEALING THE SECRETS OF HOMEOPATHIC BIOCHEMICS

DR. SWAPNA POTDAR

MD Hom, D Hom (UK)

Published by: Dr. Swapna Potdar

Pune, Maharashtra, India

Printed in India

27th October 2023

Edition:1

ISBN:978-93-6013-219-4

www.drswapnapotdar.com

DEDICATION

This book is dedicated to my husband, children and parents for their unconditional love and support all along

CONTENTS

ACKNOWLEDGMENTS

This most rewarding journey in the field of Homeopathy would not have been possible without the guidance, encouragement, and solid faith put in me by my mentors Dr. Manisha Solanki, Dr. Pradeep Sethiya, and Mrs. Latika Datar, whose depth of knowledge and wisdom continues to always inspire me. Misha Norland of the School of Homeopathy UK, and Dr. Rajan Sankaran who led the way in understanding remedies from the roots; my colleagues, students and friends, whose keen interest in constantly learning, persuaded me to write this book.

PREFACE

I have always been intrigued by the quick response of patients to Biochemics and the relative simplicity of their use. But there seemed to be a yet unexplored area of understanding them in view of the modern discoveries in medicine. Having witnessed their healing powers for about three decades, I tried to study them from their source that is, their constituent ions and correlating them to the symptoms obtained through provings. This kind of understanding gave a solid foundation to use them with great clarity in the most difficult cases, with quite miraculous results. On sharing these observations with hundreds of students and doctors, over the past decade, the knowledge was very well received, inspiring many to use this group of medicines with gratifying results. It was with their earnest persuasion that this book has come into being.

This book primarily aims at mapping the pathophysiological correlation between the Biochemic cell salts or 'Twelve Tissue salts' as they are commonly known, and their constituent ions in the body, in order to gauge their immense potential in the treatment of severe acute conditions, lingering subacutes and also incurable pathological cases.

Much has been said by Homeopaths for and against the Biochemics, the common defence being that it is polypharmacy, or that they are just so called temporary palliative remedies, which is a little unjust to their massive potential. Biochemics enable the body to respond better to any mode of treatment. How they exactly work can probably come to light in the near future, with growing research in Homeopathy.

The book is divided into chapters for convenience. But essentially there is a description of multiple cell salts in a particular chapter. So, reading the book from the beginning to the end will be much rewarding. There are case examples in every chapter to clarify and guide you to their use.

INTRODUCTION

In nature's ecosystem, we observe that there exists a mutually interdependent relationship between the animal, plant and mineral kingdom. Animals depend on other animals or plants for their food; the plants in turn depend on the soil, for water and minerals for growth. So essentially, minerals are an integral part of the three predominant natural kingdoms from where Homeopathic medicines are prepared.

Hence the importance of the twelve tissue remedies is fundamental in the treatment of patients. And we can derive great benefits from their healing potential, if we understand them in terms of the role of their constituent ions in the body.

Biochemics can be a valuable set of medicines in various challenging situations, such as -

1. Acute cases where the severity of symptoms is high;

2. In situations where there is not enough symptom clarity;

3. In incurable irreversible cases, where the vital response is weak;

4. When treating large populations in situations like pandemics;

5. Availability of the exact similimum is not possible.

But there seemed to be a pressing need, that they be understood in a modern scientific perspective so as to enable us to use them wisely and with maximum benefit to patients. This book is by no means a text book, but a means to understand the connections between the symptomatology and physiology of the Biochemics. The book describes each cell salt in a trio, for appreciating their interconnectedness.

As Homeopathy treatment is highly individualized, so is the use of Biochemics. They are actually given on the basis of a pathophysiological similarity.

1. CHAPTER ONE

The trio of inflammation

Ferrum phos, Kali mur, Calc phos

(FP KM CP)

UNDERSTANDING THE FERRUM ION

Ferrum relates to inflammatory processes, and the better way to understand its role is to study the pathophysiology of inflammation.

The body has an innate complex and well-orchestrated mechanism to rebalance and bring about harmony in its various functions. There are stimulating and inhibiting mechanisms that are so amazingly coordinated, that the human body is a miracle in itself. Self-defence is one such way to remove and annihilate the offender.

Essentially an inflammatory process is the result of an infection, an irritation, toxins, an injury or an autoimmune response. The cardinal signs of inflammation, that are 'redness, oedema, local heat, pain, and loss of function' have the purpose to bring about healing by removal of the offending factor, or the 'perceived offender' as in an autoimmune response, to clear necrotic cells, and to repair tissue.

In the first stage of inflammation, there is vasodilatation causing redness, to increase blood flow to the affected parts. This responds to the stage of Ferrum phos. Following this, epithelial cells of the blood vessels contract in response to histamine, serotonin and cytokines released from the granules of mast cells, leading to extravasation of plasma and blood cells in the extracellular space, leading to oedema. This corresponds to the stage of Kali mur.

It is the body's attempt to bring in more white blood cells, for direct attack on the offender; erythrocytes to propel more oxygen for the reactions of defence, and platelets to seal the broken tissue membranes in case of an injury. There are pro inflammatory and anti-inflammatory cytokines which optimize and harmonize this entire process. However an imbalance can lead a fatal cytokine storm or an inadequate inflammatory response on the other hand.

Ferrum phos and Kali mur aid in bringing about an optimum balance in the stimulating and inhibiting mechanisms of inflammation, in order that recovery can progress uneventfully. In a pathophysiological perspective, this means not only rapid utilization of iron or Ferrum, but also a crucial role of the calcium ions, which are responsible to bring about ion exchange between the intra and extracellular space for generation of an action potential, and the magnesium ions to activate the clotting factors.

It is actually a cascade of events as was described over two centuries ago by Schussler. Ferrum is also vital in many physiological processes. It is interesting to note that growing foetal cells have increased receptors for iron. A number of iron containing enzymes such as the cytochrome system in mitochondria, which are the energy generators of the cells, must have iron for cellular processes. So we see Ferrum phos indicated very frequently in diseases of children.

Ferrum essentially is a toxic ion and needs to be carried in a safe way by attaching to proteins such as transferrin to be taken to the cells, and also stored safely in the form of ferritin. Free iron participates in formation of free radicals and ROS (reactive oxygen species) which in excess are detrimental, and lead to neurodegenerative diseases like Alzheimer's, macular degeneration, cataract, cancer etc. Hence harmony and balance of Ferrum ions is crucial (as is also true for other ions), which can be achieved with Ferrum phos.

Iron is absorbed from food, and Ferrum phos can be helpful to improve absorption. It is important to check Ferritin levels in blood, to detect iron deficiency as the patient may have normal haemoglobin but severe symptoms of fatigue from iron deficiency. Low ferritin means low iron stores. It is a custom to use

Ferrum phos to treat iron deficiency. But is this a supplement? NO!

Ferrum phos is a potentised medicine and not a supplement, and using it on the basis of Homeopathic indications seems to harmonize ferrum ion metabolism, even in iron overload states.

Anaemia is defined as a condition in which the number of red blood cells or their oxygen carrying capacity is insufficient to meet physiological needs.

In bone marrow dysfunction, there is an impaired production of erythrocytes, and other blood cells, and not a deficiency of iron. In fact, the body absorbs more iron, in bone marrow dysfunction, due to a compensatory attempt to increase supply of iron carrying oxygen to cells. But this leads to iron overload. Infants fed with too much iron supplement, can also have an iron overload state which can be harmful. Calcarea phos is primarily needed in such situations to stimulate and support the bone marrow, Calcium ions being the initiators of all metabolic processes.

Various inflammatory conditions like rheumatoid arthritis, inflammatory bowel disease, cancer (which involves neovascularization), reduce the usable iron stores and lead to anaemic states. So Ferrum phos can be helpful in this condition as well as in cancer, to reduce its aggression.

Besides, in chronic inflammatory conditions, there is a reduced erythropoietin stimulation of the bone marrow, leading to impaired production of healthy erythrocytes. Ferrum phos with Calcarea phos can be helpful here.

As we now relate Ferrum phos to congestion, and inflammation, it is worthwhile to note here that in CKD or chronic renal disease, the compromised number of functional nephrons results in intra renal hypertension to compensate for the reduced renal function. This unfortunately leads to further damage of nephrons. Ferrum phos reduces this intra renal congestion, and helps to preserve the renal function, along with Calcarea phos and Natrum salts, as indicated. This has been later elaborated with a case example.

In summary, we see that iron has many more crucial roles in addition of being the oxygen carrier in Haemoglobin. Using Ferrum phos at the beginning of inflammation effectively helps to do the required job without having to escalate the pro inflammatory factors.

To summarize Ferrum Phos (FP)-

1. First stage of inflammation, dusky redness.

2. Aggression/ restlessness.

3. Dryness/ inflammation of vagina.

4. Congestion/ haemorrhage, e.g. epistaxis, colitis.

5. All kinds of pain-as it is usually a sign of inflamma-tion.

6. Fever with headache and red eyes, photophobia.

7. Enuresis from worms (Also NP SIL) – Deworming FP NP 12X.

8. Summer / sun <<.

9.*Useful in iron deficiency anaemia/low Haemoglobin count. NOT in low RBC count.

*Here Use Calc Phos.

10. FP in a powder form applied to open wounds, and ulcers helps rapid healing.

Understanding with some case examples-

1. Tonsillitis-A five years old boy was brought in with fever 101^0F, throbbing pain and heat of the head, inability to swallow from pricking pain. On examination, his tonsils were enlarged, bright red and had 2 mm dots of pus pockets. He would take only liquid and warm food, with difficulty. These episodes occurred every time the weather changed from hot to cold or hot to rainy.

The first dose was Calcarea phos 200X, 2 tabs (A/F change of weather) followed by FPCPKM 30X, 5 tablets each in 150 ml of water, 10 ml every 2 hours, along with Belladonna 30C.The recovery was quick in a day and the second day the pain and discomfort was forgotten.

Similarly the indicated remedy maybe Hepar sulph, or Phytolacca, or any other, and the case can well be treated with just that. But when symptoms are not very well marked, or the remedy is not available, **Biochemics are versatile enough to start the healing, on the basis of the pathophysiological phenomenon occurring in the case**.

2. They are a boon to Homeopathy in pandemic situations, where you can start to help people even before a genus epidemicus can be decided upon. And that certainly helped tremendously in the COVID pandemic.

FP CP KM 30X were administered to 6000 people during the pandemic and they were monitored through group representatives. Where there was a chance I indivisualised the cases and administered the indicated acute remedy in the centicimal potency, along with the Biochemics. The outcome was extremely rewarding with very few casualties, milder symptoms, and rapid recovery in the moderate to severe cases. Results have been published in Hpathy.

https://hpathy.com/scientific-research/a-retrospective-study-to-evaluate-the-safety-and-efficacy-of-homoeopathic-prophylaxis-in-ncovid19-with-tuberculinum-aviaire-and-homeopathic-remedies/

When the vital reaction is weak or the infective pathogen is too virulent, measures to support the life force can greatly alleviate suffering. We understand Biochemics in this manner, to support the body's own mechanisms to improve treatment outcomes. The indicated Homeopathic remedy in the centicimal potency will act faster and better when the tissues are supported with the tissue salts.

3. Recurrent infections-

If every change in weather triggers a cold, throat irritation, and cough with or without fever, the indicated constitutional Homeopathy medicine, can be given infrequently but cell salts Ferrum Phos, Calcarea phos, Kali mur, given one tablet daily for a month can dramatically have faster and better outcome. It is found that the 6X potency can be used when secretions are scanty, but the 30X is better when secretions are more marked. This is a clinical observation.

4. Gastroenteritis-

Gastritis, with or without enteritis, with vomiting of anything eaten, or diarrhoea, indicates an inflammation of the lining mucus membranes, and can usually be associated with dehydration, hypotension, or fever. A rapid improvement can be achieved with consideration of these pathophysiological phenomena, and giving Ferrum phos, Kali mur,(both for the inflammation) Natrum mur, Kali phos and Calc Phos (restoratives and electrolyte balancers) in the 6X potency one tablet each, every one hour along with the indicated Homeopathic remedy, bring about recovery in a few hours. This has been elaborated later in the chapter on Natrum mur.

KALI MUR (KM)

The cell salt that naturally follows Ferrum phos, or is even needed along with Ferrum phos is Kali mur or potassium chloride in the potentised form. And that potentised form is different from the chemical having its own special characters determined by drug proving.

Kali mur relates to the second stage of inflammation, i.e. of exudation of plasma in the intercellular space. So the first stage is congestion where there is vasodilatation, causing redness and pain from the irritated nerve endings and the pressure of more blood on the affected tissue. The mast cells then release the cytokines, serotonin and histamine, causing endothelial cells to separate and help extravasation of plasma into the tissue or through the serous/mucus membranes. This is where Kali mur is needed. Serous discharges, swelling, albuminous secretions, formation of fibrin, liver functions are the predominant areas of action of Kali mur.

Kali mur is indicated in the following:

1. Second stage of inflammation with exudations, and swelling.

2. Whiteness is a theme of KM - white albuminous discharges.

3. Useful in many conditions of the ear due to its affinity for the ear.

4. Relates to fibrin; can prevent clotting due to its action of harmonizing function of fibrin formation.

Thus in thrombosis, both Deep Vein Thrombosis (DVT) / and Superficial Vein Thrombosis (SVT) the use of FP CP KM CF 6X has proven to be rewarding, evidenced by dissolution of the thrombus, confirmed on Doppler studies. Here Calcarea Fluor (CF) relates to the degenerative nature of atherosclerosis that is usually present with thrombosis.

5. Kali mur is useful in albuminuria, considering that the cause usually is related to an inflammatory/degenerative process in the kidneys.

6. As a complementary medicine for meningitis, along with the indicated medicine.

7. Ferrum phos and Kali mur are important in treating avascular necrosis, macular degeneration, and in conditions of reduced blood perfusion to tissues.

8. Kali mur 6X applied locally to a wound or ulcer, helps formation of healthy granulation tissue.

9. Kali mur follows Ferrum Phos, and is followed by Kali sulph.

CALCAREA PHOS (CP)

Calcarea phos is the third cell salt in the trio of inflammation with FP KM. KS also, is valuable in the secretory stage of resolution of inflammation, and has been described in the chapter on the sulphuris'. In order to appreciate the importance of Calcarea phos, we need to understand the role of calcium and phosphate ions in the body.

UNDERSTANDING CALCIUM IONS

Life begins with a surge of calcium ions when the embryo is formed. So that is the centre stage that Calcium ions deserve in our study.

In the early 1880s Sydney Ringer, a British physician and physiologist in London, was studying the beating of an isolated frog heart outside of the body. He hoped to identify the substances that would allow the isolated heart to beat normally for a time. Distilled water was being used to keep it immersed, but one day by mistake tap water was used instead, and the frog heart started beating! On investigating further, it was discovered that tap water in London was high in Calcium. And this is how Ringer's lactate was eventually discovered.

Calcium is the most abundant mineral in the body. It binds to protein molecules, and makes them functional. E.g. clotting factors. These are completely functionless without presence of calcium ions in the right proportion.

The slightest decrease of calcium ions in plasma cause voltage gated sodium (Na) ion channels to leak sodium ions into nerve cells, making them hyper excitable, leading to spasms, tetany, and paraesthesia. Increase in calcium ions leads to more calcium bound to sodium channels, causing lethargy, constipation, and LABILE EMOTIONS. So we now see the interconnected functions of the calcium and natrum ions.

Calcium ions are low inside the cells. They act as messengers in muscle contractions, and release of hormones, like insulin from beta cells, or neurotransmitters like acetyl choline and in cardiac muscle contraction. So we see now why Calcarea phos has spasms, cramps, numbness, and myopathy.

The calcium ion is vital to normal, harmonious cell metabolism. Minor imbalance causes imbalance in the sodium and potassium ions, leading to a cascade of events resulting in disease.

So we see that-

1. Calcium is involved in all cellular metabolic processes.

2. It is present in the extra cellular fluid where it helps in maintaining structure as in the skeleton.

3. In the cell, it acts as a signalling ion.

4. Excess calcium inhibits parathyroid hormone and 1, 25(OH) 2D (Vitamin D), the latter being responsible for intestinal calcium absorption.

5. Excess of sodium or salt in the diet leads to calciuria, and can cause formation of renal calculus. We find therefore Calcarea phos and Natrum Mur indicated for renal calculi.

So we understand here that without an optimum level of calcium ions all metabolic and tissue functions could be disrupted, and thus calcium ions have the importance in our body functions like the 'zero' has in mathematics!

PHOSPHATE IONS

They are present in every cell and give structure and strength to the tissues with calcium. Phosphate ions are required for various biochemical processes, including energy production and pH regulation. Phosphorus in it acts as a buffer to neutralize acids.

Natrum phos has a buffer like action to balance the acidity of secretions. Phosphate ions fuel energy with adenosine triphosphate (ATP).

To summarize Calcarea Phos-

1. It is the central remedy in Biochemistry. A precursor to others.

2. A disturbance in the calcium ions leads to disturbance of other ions.

3. After Calc phos all other indicated medicines act better and 'hold' well.

4. Needed for rapidly growing cells. Bone marrow, bones, teeth, hair.

5. Rickety children/rickety adults (Patients of diabetes mellitus, cancer, chronic debilitating diseases).

6. A restorative in states of depletion, such as loss of vital fluids.

7. Physiologically stressful phases like-delayed milestones, growth spurt/growing pains, puberty, pregnancy, delivery, lactation, second childhood (old age).

8. Headache during the secondary teething phase.

9. Ailments from grief, disappointed love, sexual excess, weather changes.

10. Worse in damp cold weather.

11. First remedy in cold. Single dose CP 200X, followed by the indicated medicines, will give much better results.

12. Ailments from change of weather.

13. Irascible anger from contradiction. Paralyzed felt as if-walk with a limp when furious.

14. Anxiety about health/ health of others.

15. Development of children arrested/very slow. Hence useful in autism.

16. Lymphadenopathy.

17. Delusions-away from home and must get there.

18. Lascivious, nymphomania. Masturbation in children-girls-Calc phos 200X. (Boys- Aur, Plat)

19. RESTLESSNESS, wander desire to. Constantly desires change. Therefore useful in ADHD, restless

leg syndrome, restless adolescents, and adults who behave like adolescents.

20. Averse to rules / doing what is told.

21. Live on loans. Spend thrifts. Like to always dress well, in dot patterns (CP, Phos, Sep)

22. Addictions. Calc phos helps to reduce the uncontrollable cravings.

23. Headache of school children-CP and MP

24. Pain in abdomen on eating - Clinically verified

25. Calcarea phos has been extensively used, rather abused as a calcium supplement. But we need to remember that this is a potentised, dynamised medicine, which has a wide range of action. It certainly can improve calcium metabolism, and absorption, but must not be used unless the patient's symptoms indicate it.

Here is a Case to understand the brilliant Biochemics working-

A CASE OF Chronic Kidney Disease (CKD)

A male patient 'Mr.JM' with dark skin, medium built, and large suffused watery eyes, with unkempt, dry grey and wavy hair, aged 67 years, came in walking with great anxiety and uncertainty, exclaiming at every step, with the diagnosis of CKD.

His S.Creatinine 3.9 ug/dl (normal range 0.7-1.3 mg/dl), S. Potassium 5.7 mEq/L (normal 3.6 to 5.2 mEq/L) eGFR 40 ml/min (normal above 60-80 ml/Min), Blood pressure 150/100 mm Hg (normal 120-130/80-90 mm Hg)

He had suffered a hypertensive stroke on the right side, a few years back. He walked with a lot of struggle, terrified at taking a step lest he would fall, and obstinately refusing to use a walking device for support. His speech was barely audible and indistinct. He had been diagnosed with chronic renal failure stage 3, which includes a range of GFR between 30-59, indicating moderate reduction in renal function.

This also meant that we needed to act quickly, and effectively to try to prevent him from deteriorating to severe degree of CKD. In such situations the Biochemics support cellular function in the functional renal cells and help the patient's organs to respond better to the indicated constitutional remedy.

He was accompanied by his wife, who spoke on his behalf, and shared that he was very impatient, and wanted things immediately. He would keep on pestering till he got what he wanted.

His behaviour was very childlike, dependent on his wife for everything, and not willing to cooperate in most activities. He loved chocolates and would want to have at least one daily in spite of his diabetes, which was luckily in control. He was very obstinate, and wouldn't do something he did not want to. Not fear but, TERROR of falling, wants to be held. As if sure that he will fall when he stands or walks. He was rubbing his face with his palms frequently. Let's see the repertorisation-

Mind; carried desires to be- Bor, Gels, Brom, Sulph, Bry, Calc, Ant-t, Cham

Clinging; grasps at others- Bor, Gels, Cupr

Mind; FEAR falling of,carried being- Bor, Gels

Face; cobweb sensation Bor, Brom,Sulph, Bry, Calc

So you may notice that we consider his prominent characteristic individualizing symptoms, and not the pathological symptoms like renal failure etc. In support of Borax 200C which was given as a weekly dose, Calc phos 6X, Ferrum Phos 6X, Kali mur 6X, Natrum mur 6X, Natrum sulph 6X and Kali phos 6X are all the Biochemics needed for him.

Let's see why-

Calcarea phos (CP)-the basic cell salt without which, cellular metabolism cannot be improved. Other remedies act better and hold well after Calc phos.

Ferrum phos (FP)-CKD implies destruction of a considerable number of nephrons, which means the body needs the remaining healthier nephrons to work more. Due to this there is development of intra renal hypertension, in the body's attempt to increase blood flow and improve filtration. This is actually detrimental to the remaining nephrons, leading to further damage. FP helps reduce this congestion and preserve renal function to a great extent.

Kali mur (KM) - Albuminuria is a symptom of Kali mur and CKD causes albuminuria. The excretion of albumin is in itself detrimental to nephrons, leading to further damage. Kali mur can improve this by virtue of the pathophysiological symptom similarity.

Natrum mur(NM) and Kali phos(KP) - Electrolyte imbalance is part of the pathophysiology of CKD. Atrial natriuretic peptide and renal aldosterone help maintain sodium ion balance and therefore the fluid and electrolyte balance in a healthy body. But in CKD this function is compromised, leading to water retention, and increase in serum sodium and potassium. More sodium in blood can cause increased hypertension, which is detrimental to CKD and more serum potassium can lead to dangerous arrhythmias. Thus these high levels of sodium and potassium are associated with increased mortality in CKD patients.

Natrum mur helps sodium ion balance in tissues, and potassium ion balance can be well achieved with Kali phos.

Natrum Sulph (NS) - This cell salt has an affinity for kidneys and improves and supports renal function.

Why 6X - This is more of a clinical observation that the 6X potency stimulates tissue function in irreversible pathology more effectively, than the higher which are more subtle and relate to a higher energy frequency.

So this way we need to understand what exactly is happening in the patient's body in terms of the pathophysiology of the disease, and select the required cell salt so that we can save the patient from further deterioration.

Mr. JM was given Borax 200 as weekly doses and FP KM CP NM NS KP all 6x on alternate days 1 tablet each, for a month. The first improvement was reduced blood pressure, improvement in his energy levels, reduction in anxiety, reduction in serum creatinine to 3.0mg/dl from 3.9 mg/dl; serum potassium came down to 5.5 mEq/L from 5.7 mEq/L. He was monitored every month, and there was a gradual improvement in him and his renal function. At this point I tried to discontinue the Biochemics for him, and continued only with the Homeopathic medicine that was indicated that time, in weekly doses. I found that his S.Creatinine levels began to rise, and also his potassium. I therefore resumed the Biochemic regimen as a supportive.

In about a year, he was able to speak much more clearly, and had improvement in the strength in his limbs. He was so very grateful for the miracle of Homeopathy, that he was most earnest to visit the clinic. He lived well for another 7 years, and never needed a dialysis.

2. CHAPTER TWO

The electrolyte and nerve balancers

Kali phos, Mag Phos, Natrum Mur

(KP MP NM)

UNDERSTANDING KALI PHOS (KP)

Potassium phosphate (K_2HPO_4) is prepared by adding potassium carbonate and dilute phosphoric acid. Potassium depletion in the body leads to neurological dysfunction, and here we see why there exists a strong affinity of Kali phos for the nervous system.

As Hahnemann rightly said, Kali phos if well studied, could empty the mental asylums. It certainly is not a panacea for mental illnesses but has its own special characters.

1. Exhaustion, depression, senile dementia, fear of noises, fear of future, lack of will, brain fag, blankness, staring.

2. Offensiveness, cadaverous odour

3. Blackness; blackish secretions and discharges

4. Sepsis

5. Cancer

6. Dry gangrene

7. Burning pains

In all of the above numbered symptoms that most books mention, we see that Kali phos is a deep acting remedy having a destructive pathology, implying the syphillitic miasm of Hahnemann. So many times it is used quite casually for anxiety or stress, in frequent and large doses, by which I mean 4 tablets 4 times a day, without understanding its vast potential.

This book is meant to bridge the gap between why these symptoms are present in the remedy and how we can use them effectively. And we could best learn this with a case.

CASE OF JONTY-the dog

Jonty was a black handsome labrador. Very much loved and pampered by his family. He enjoyed being the centre of attention and affection. But I got a distress call one day saying that he is desperately ill, in the hospital, passing blood in his vomit and black tarry stools. Nothing seemed to be working, and he already was on IV antibiotics, and supportive treatment. His vitals were collapsing fast.

It was our last chance to try and save him. His brief history revealed that few days back, there came a golden retriever pup in the house. And all the focus suddenly shifted to the pup. Jonty was terribly upset and offended. He would bark and wail, and refused food and drink. He started losing weight, and developed diarrhoea, which got worse and here he was now.

You see this is a desperate situation. His vital reaction is weakening by the minute. We need to act fast and effectively. My first dose was Ignatia 50M, followed by Arsenicum album 6C with Calc phos 6X, Kali Phos 6X and Ferrum Phos 6X, 3 tablets every 20 minutes. Animals need more number of pills and also they respond quickly to Homeopathy; this is my clinical observation.

The family followed this meticulously. Why three remedies? The reason is an understanding of the body's fine orchestration of ion functions, which indicate the required Biochemics.

Ignatia 50M as the first dose, because we got this history of emotional shock, which started the whole problem. That is the core of the issue.

Arsenicum Album 6C, as the vital reaction is deteriorating, and centicimal potencies act faster than decimal or X potencies. Ars alb relates to offensiveness, severe gastroenteritis, and collapse. So Ars alb 6C repeated every half hour.

Calcarea phos 6X as the body needs support to step up the failing cellular metabolism,

Kali phos 6X, because it confirms with blackish offensive secretions, and collapse.

Ferrum Phos 6X, because there are signs of severe inflammation all along the gastro intestinal tract.

Jonty revived in 3-4 hours. He was stable and sent home to live a jolly happy life of 17 years, without the new pup! If we can save a life this way so be it!

It is appropriate here to understand what role potassium has in the body.

KALIUM /POTASSIUM ION-

Almost all the ingested potassium is excreted by the kidneys and through stools. The body maintains a potassium level between 3.5 to 5.0 mM which is largely intracellular. Large scale tissue damage can lead to massive hyperkalemia especially as in such situations, there is acute kidney injury and reduced potassium excretion as well.

Rapid tumour lysis, acidosis, congestive cardiac failure, volume depletion, diabetes, diabetic nephropathy, chronic kidney disease, HIV, disseminated fungal infections, tuberculosis, autoimmune, connective tissue disorders, metastatic cancer and even old age, are some causes of hyperkalemia, which is a level above 5.5 mM .

In these pathologies, symptoms of Kali phos can usually be found, like extreme exhaustion, offensive secretions, blackish discolouration of body surfaces or of secretions, and hypotension or collapse. So Kali phos can be a great support to the weak life force.

It's all a study of the ion functions in the body!

1. Paralysis in hyperthyroidism also called TPP (thyrotoxic periodic paralysis) is due to hypokalemia.

2. Also endogenous secretion of insulin due to carbohydrate load or exogenous insulin can provoke hypokalemia. We need to understand here that, this is why diabetic patients can be helped with Kali phos.

Hering had found that Kali phos causes glycosuria, hence useful in diabetes. In diabetes, we have a metabolically stressful state. The body cannot utilize the sugar for energy. Exhaustion, weight loss, infections, nervousness are common symptoms of diabetes. Degenerative pathologies, like retinal detachment, recurrent infections, cardiomyopathy, kidney disease, hyperkalemia are concerning complications. Kali phos being a deep acting remedy can be of great help in diabetes. It can support the action of the constitutional remedy or rather, will help the body to respond better and prevent many of the complications of diabetes.

But remember, not too many doses, but minimum, just enough to elicit a response. Or you end up causing what you are trying to prevent. And this applies to all our Homeopathic remedies, especially the Bio-chemics.

3. Sympathetic nervous system alterations can cause hypokalemia. Which means stressful states, head injury, myocardial infarction, and also too much of dietary caffeine.

4. Kali phos has saved the emotional trauma of so many toddlers and their anxious mothers, when they both suffer separation anxiety at the beginning of school. Separation anxiety of students, who move away from home for the first time. Or so many such situations where it seems that it is impossible to deal with things. The mind is clouded and exhausted, incapable of functioning. Kali phos 200X 2 tablets only once. And that is the miracle. 'The single dose miracle'.

5. So do we now find the situations when we can use Kali phos, and also why Hahnemann advised avoiding stimulants. As stimulants contain caffeine, which can deplete serum potassium.

6. In the body, hypokalemia is invariably accompanied by hypophosphatemia and hypomagnesemia. This sheds light on the interconnectedness of Kali phos, and Mag phos.

7. Diarrhoea causes hypokalemia. So we use Kali phos here in many intestinal pathologies like inflammatory bowel disease (IBD), coeliac disease, and also laxative abuse with brilliant results.

8. Cushing's syndrome or use of glucocorticoids causes hypokalemia.

9. In general hypokalemia causes arrhythmias, heart failure, skeletal myopathy, and paralysis of intestinal muscles or ileus, acute kidney injury, renal cysts, risk of hypertension and stroke.

10. Kali phos is indicated in impaired potassium ion balance. So in both hyperkalemia and hypokalemia, Kali phos can be helpful to restore the balance of potassium and significantly improve prognosis. But in every case try to understand the underlying pathology, and choose the required Biochemic salt accordingly, and then watch the amazing benefits to the patient.

MAG PHOS (MP)

UNDERSTANDING MAGNESIUM IONS

Magnesium is the second most abundant element inside human cells, and is second only to calcium ions. Magnesium ions regulate over 300 biochemical reactions in the body through their role as enzyme co-factors, including generation of ATP. Magnesium is necessary for lipid metabolism and to adjust the levels of cholesterol produced and released into the blood stream.

Magnesium is needed to produce energy. An imbalance in magnesium would lead to our muscles being in a permanent state of contraction. We see here the correlation that homeopathic Mag phos has symptoms like cramps, spasmodic affections. This understanding can be applied to many organs. Abdominal cramps, menstrual colic, bronchial spasms. Mag phos is helpful with other tissue salts like Ferrum phos and Kali mur in bronchospasm of bronchial asthma, and bronchitis.

Ferrum Phos and Kali mur help to reduce the inflammation, and Mag phos will relieve the bronchospasm to give better and quicker relief in chest infections, and congestions.

In ureteric colic the smooth muscles of the ureter contract from the irritation of the calculus, and there is also an inflammatory reaction. Here Ferrum phos, helps to reduce inflammation, Calcarea phos helps to fragment the calculus, and Mag phos helps release the ureteric smooth muscle spasm, to finally expel it with ease.

Magnesium ions are a content of the white matter of nervous tissue. And Mag phos is a princely remedy in optic neuritis, trigeminal neuralgia, and sciatica. Mag phos helps severe shooting lancinating pain, better by warm applications, and heat.

Mag phos is helpful in obstruction of urine, due to its action of relieving smooth muscle contraction.

CASE OF ACUTE URINE RETENTION

I had an elderly patient who called in great distress as he was unable to pass urine though his bladder was full. What happened was, he was on a long bus journey, and the bus wouldn't stop for many hours at a stretch. He got into trouble with the driver, who was rude and non-cooperative. Luckily he was carrying some Biochemic medicines for first aid, and I advised him to take 3 tablets of Mag phos 30X with warm water every 15 minutes. Two doses relieved his agony. That is the magic of Homeopathy. The 'Two dose magic!'

Summarising Mag Phos-

1. Mag phos people are hurried, and keep moving things from one place to another. They must move fast. So it is useful in Attention Deficit Hyperactivity Disorder (ADHD) and Autism Spectrum Disorder with Kali phos and Calc Phos , to achieve better and faster results with the indicated constitutional remedy.

2. Repeats same complaints over and over and gets hiccoughs during. Hiccoughs as we know are spasmodic contractions of the diaphragm.

3. Recurrent headaches of school children,

4. Disorders of the nervous system,

5. Epilepsy,

6. Cramps and spasms.

7. WORKS BEST WHEN GIVEN IN HOT WATER

The five phos i.e. Mag phos, Natrum phos, Kali phos, Ferrum phos, Calcarea phos, are used together for senile weakness, or conditions of weak vital reaction, cancer cachexia, and anaemia. But the selection needs to always be based upon the indications; the patho-physiological similarity is the secret to achieve the miracle cure!

NATRUM MUR (NM)

UNDERSTANDING THE SODIUM AND CHLORIDE ION

Sodium and chloride ions are vital for electrolyte and water balance of the body. Sodium chloride ions pull water with them. So plants that are grown in soil containing more salt wither away. The colloid osmotic pressure in the extra cellular fluid is maintained by the sodium ions .Chloride ions are typically always reabsorbed with sodium ions to maintain homeostasis of osmolality between the intra and extracellular fluid . So Natrum mur is important in achieving fluid and electrolyte balance.

Sodium ions are responsible for carrying nutrients to cells and carrying waste products away from cells. Something like the nurturing action of a mother. Here we can see why the themes of 'mother' are related to the Natrum group of remedies. The nervous system contributes to water and electrolyte balance in an important way.

Vasopressin is synthesized in the neurons within the hypothalamus, and released through the axons that extend into the posterior pituitary or neurohypophysis. Vasopressin or Anti diuretic hormone (ADH) helps promote water reabsorption in the kidneys, and thus maintain the osmotic pressure in the body. We note here that Kali phos has an active role in the nervous system.

There is also a network of osmoreceptor neurons which sense the changes in osmolality and release vasopressin that leads to signals of increased thirst and reabsorption of sodium and fluid, in hypvolemia, and the reverse in hypervolemia.

In our understanding of the Biochemics we now can see the close relationship between the sodium, chloride and potassium ions, and thus the link between Kali phos and Natrum mur. Hence many times Natrum mur, and Kali phos follow each other or may be needed together.

1. In gastroenteritis FP KM CP NM KP 6X all in equal proportions e.g. 5 tablets each in 150 ml (1 tea cup) of water, 10 ml (2 tsp) every 45 minutes can bring the symptoms in control in a few hours when given along with the indicated remedy. The recovery is faster, appetite is restored and the patient recovers from the episode with very little weakness.

And here is why-

Ferrum phos- as there is an inflammatory process in the gut;

Kali mur- there is profuse exudation causing diarrhoea;

Calcarea phos- the primary ion needed for optimum function of other ions;

Natrum mur- as there is water and electrolyte imbalance in diarrhoea that has to be corrected;

Kali phos- Weakness, due to low potassium in diarrhoea.

Is it not quite straight and simple!

2.In premenopausal women reduction in oestrogen and progesterone can lead to a relatively hyponatraemic state causing some degree of oedema in the brain due to increased activity of the sodium potassium pump which otherwise stays inhibited . So we see many symptoms in Natrum mur related to the menstrual cycle. Premenstrual syndrome, headaches, migraine related to the hormone cycle, finds a wonderful remedy in Natrum mur when symptoms match.

3. Natrum mur relates to cysts. Ovarian cysts, and renal cysts. And this is due to the property of sodium chloride of attracting water. An imbalance of natrum and chloride ions leads to the cysts not resolving naturally. PCOS is being accepted as a multisystem disorder, as modern medicine now appreciates the more holistic nature of diseases. It relates to imbalances starting at the hypothalamus, and the neurohypophysis presenting as cysts in the ovaries. This correlates to the Homeopathic holistic approach of considering the PNEI psycho-neuro-endocrino-immunological axis in ALL cases.

4. Natrum mur is helpful in granulomas or 'proud flesh' which means excessive granulation tissue, impairing apposition of the edges of the wound thus delaying healing.

CASE OF 'Episiotomy granuloma' or EG:

A lady aged 24 yrs. just delivered her 2nd baby girl, 15 days ago came with an EG. She said to me "No one was supportive for my pregnancy so I decided that I will not take anyone's help after delivery. While getting up from the bed, I slid. I didn't realise that something may have gone wrong, except when I went for a follow up. The gynaecologist discovered this granuloma. She adviced to apply Calendula cream, which I did, thrice a day. But no effect. She wants me to get admitted again and plans to scrape and re suture. I don't want to go back to hospital again."

The rubrics that I thought important in her case were-

1. Indignation during pregnancy-Nat Mur

Indignation-Anger mingled with disdain, extreme anger, and effects of anger

Disdain: haughtiness, pride, arrogance

2. Granulations – Nat mur, Sil are the two prominent remedies amongst the Biochemics listed in repertories.

I could notice that she did not have any other com-plaints, and also that she was lactating. I decided to apply Nat mur 6X powder of 1 tab locally, as I felt that a higher potency given orally was not needed and also that would not act quickly on the granuloma.

To my greatest wonder and disbelief, the next day there was 50% reduction in size, of the lesion, and it totally disappeared on the 5th day.

That, I call the magic of the Biochemics! A single remedy, and minimum dose. Needless to say, the gy-naecologist became a staunch follower of Homeopa-thy!

To summarize Natrum Mur (NM):

1. NM relates to water filled cysts-renal, ovarian.

2. Granulations.

3. Hypertension – FP CP NM KP 6X solution (5 tabs each in 150 ml water, 2 tsp (10 ml) frequent intervals).

4. Dehydration FP KM CP NM 6X, 4 tabs in 150 ml 10ml 1hourly.

5. Premenstrual Syndrome

6. Hydramnios

7. Glaucoma, Cataract- (CF, SIL)

8. Arrythmia; misses every 4th beat.

9. Renal calculi, renal failure

10. MIND- (in brief)

Tears from eyes when laughing.

Immoderate laughter.

Want to be alone for days.

Delusion looks wretched.

Feels she is pitied and frets more.

Consolation aggravates.

Takes everything in a bad part.

Dwells on past disagreeable offences.

3. CHAPTER THREE

The infection, hyperacidity, and deformity healers

SILICEA, NATRUM PHOS AND CALCAREA FLUOR (SIL NP CF)

UNDERSTANDING SILICEA

A Homoeopath's famous surgical knife, and antibiotic. Silicea has won many laurels for draining out pus from abscesses and lumps. The indications here are a tender painful lump, well, 'tender' most of the time.

CASE OF A SEBACEOUS CYST

In my early days of practice, I had my professor come to me for the treatment of a sebaceous cyst. The cyst was on his back, about two inches long and one inch thick. It looked unsightly to his wife, but otherwise caused no pain or discomfort. He told me that the operation had already been planned and that he just wanted to see what I could do with it with my Homeopathy! He asked me several questions like, what would happen after taking the medicines? How long would it take? What would happen of the cyst wall? And so on.. My answer was that, 'Homeopathic medicines will stimulate the inflammatory process and help the contents of his cyst to drain out. The cyst wall would remain back, and that there are chances of it becoming painful during this process'.

It was a viva voce isn't it? And many patients certainly want to know what to expect.

I gave him three tablets of Silicea 200X, and requested that he come back in a week. He didn't come back in a week, and I thought maybe he had his surgery. But he came two months later with another colleague, who needed treatment.

"What happened of the sebaceous cyst?' I asked him. "Oh yes! I forgot to update you. I was travelling and it got swollen and inflamed, formed a soft point, and burst when I was asleep. Yes, it was painful that day, but then it drained and I gently cleaned it. No surgery needed!'

That was a moment of ecstasy as I was quite new in the field then! And from then on the trust in homeopathy got a push in their hospital in a big way! Here again did we not see the 'single dose miracle'!

To SUMMARIZE SILICEA

1. It promotes inflammation and pus formation by stimulating the WBCs. Abscess, Sebaceous cysts, pustular tonsillitis are the home ground of Silicea.

2. Silicea can expel foreign bodies from the soft tissues, so use cautiously in patients who have mesh implants for their hernia.

3. Malabsorption is another important character of Silicea. This could mean lack of food, or of nutritious food, or the inability to absorb it. Silicea patients have weak nails, and bones.

4. Lack of reaction, or sluggishness of reactions.

5. Bad effects of vaccination. This throws light on a very wide range of problems like Autism, ADHD, Aspergers, Autism spectrum disorder, chronic eczema, the list is endless. This is an area of controversy, as there are no proved evidences of a correlation between vaccination and the above disorders. Nevertheless, when many parents share that they started to notice changes in the child's behaviour, after vaccines, Silicea in the higher potencies, like 1M, LM, have shown to start improvement.

5. Osteomyelitis. Silicea gives wonderful results, by stimulating the body's immune mechanisms to eliminate the infection.

6. Primary or secondary sterility when the constitutional symptoms match. When the cause is adhesions in the fallopian tubes, Silicea and Kali mur may help to restore patency of the tubes.

7. Silicea people are very obstinate, headstrong. It is difficult to make them give in. They may appear very

shy, as they worry about what people may think of them, or that they may be laughed at. They are sensitive about their social image. A/F egotism is a prominent rubric of Silicea. This again confirms the theme of the high regard for themselves and their self-esteem. There is another pole to Silicea of being faint hearted and diffident, but do you see why; it is the overwhelming fear of hurt to their social image.

8. Silicea has offensive and profuse sweat, and feet become sore from the sweat, like Graphitis.

9. I would definitely advice to *Avoid use of Silicea in gastroenteritis *, as it can aggravate the diarrhoea.

10. I would also advice to be very cautious when using Silicea in ureteric calculus, as it can often lead to pyuria, or pus in the ureter. Silicea like other Homeopathic remedies can cause what it can cure. It can cause pus and it can cure pus you see!

This book does not intend to list out all the symptoms, but its purpose is to shed light on the underlying wisdom of the Biochemics.

NATRUM PHOS (NP)

It has a marked acridity of secretions, which are thick yellow.

A CASE OF HYPERACIDITY

I had a patient who came to me for weight loss and acid like secretions. He complained in an agitated, 'acidic' tone that, "No doctor is able to understand that I pour out acid from my gut. The moment I eat anything, the acid starts to burn in my abdomen, and in no time I have to go to pass stool. It burns the parts, and my inner wear has also got holes from the acidic secretions. The hospital sends me away saying that this is not possible, as so much acid would first ulcerate my bowels! I can bring my clothes to show you how they get holes though they are new. I am also losing weight, as all that I eat passes out in no time".

1. Acidic nature of discharges, and an acidic attitude to it, the grand generalization holds true you see!

His tongue was coated golden yellow at the base, like the text book symptom of Natrum Phos. And he got Natrum phos 30X 1 tablet twice a day for a month. A changed man came back saying that he has gained half kilogram of weight, and his inner wear is not holed this time!

2. Natrum phos relates to too much lactic acid in the blood, i.e. too much sugar in the blood. So in diabetes mellitus, Natrum phos will help better metabolism of sugar, and improved insulin production with the help of Calcarea phos. The role of Kali phos in diabetes mellitus has been described earlier.

3. Natrum Phos is a wonderful deworming agent. It is a pH corrector, and will help to expel worms from the body with Ferrum phos, as there usually exists a subclinical inflammation in such situations. Natrum phos 12X and Ferrum phos 12X two tablets of each once a week for four weeks acts as a great deworming agent. I have used this extensively in animals as well, with double the number of tablets mentioned above, i.e. four tablets of each, with great results.

I cannot conclude Natrum phos without the story of a very busy doctor, who was so fiercely independent, and wanted to always eat out. She never had her meals on time, nor ate the healthy type of food. "I know I shouldn't be eating all this. But I can't just keep away from the pastries, and the tangy spices. I have had such severe episodes of pain in my abdomen, and got diagnosed with ulcerative gastritis. I still sometimes feel like there is a dragon in me spitting fire. I get pain in my abdomen, as if there was a snake biting me. Please don't tell me my mistakes, because I know. Just help me with this somehow."

Natrum phos and Ferrum phos 6X one tablet each, every 2 hours put to rest the dragon and snake in a few hours. She now uses them as and when needed.

We sometimes make things complicated though they can be solved easily. Isn't it?

CALCAREA FLUOR (CF)

Calcium ions and fluoride ions need to be understood to appreciate how we can use Calcarea fluor more effectively.

Fluoride is an ion required in small amounts 0.5 to 10 mg daily. It is easily obtained from water, tea, coffee, milk, wheat, yogurt, cheese, apples, avocado, chicken, raisins, etc. Fluoride is known to be related to strength of bones, and the teeth. Excess can lead to fluorosis, with staining of teeth and is usually not serious.

We have spoken at length about the role of calcium ions, and here it is worth repeating that calcium ions are needed for growth and strength of the skeleton as well as all cellular metabolic processes.

1. Calcarea fluor relates to bony growths. Spur formation, osteophytes, indicating an imbalance between the osteoblastic and osteoclastic activity. I have seen good results with the 6X frequently like daily for few months, or 12X weekly. The susceptibility and sensitivity will decide between 6X and 12X. 12X for the more sensitive patients.

Calcarea Fluor seems to bring about the balance so that osteoclasts begin to remodel the bone, and slow down the degenerative process. Hopefully research in the near future will shed light to explain this phenomenon that has been verified numerous times in clinical practice.

2. Stony hardness is another characteristic for Calcarea fluor. Stony hard tumours and glands. Hence in cancer, CF may help to improve chances of slowing down the activity of cancer cells. 200X would be advisable weekly or every 15 days, to match the severity of the case.

3. Keratosis, painful callosities, soften with use of Calcarea fluor. Use the 6X repeatedly for a month or more.

4. Varicose veins, aneurysms, find a wonderful help in Calc fluor. It will help reduce the congestion of varicosity and prevent ulcer formation. Its relation to the elastic fibres in tissues could be the reason for achieving this. I have used the 6X frequently or the 12X

weekly once for few months in such cases with great benefit to the patients.

5. Crooked nails, crooked looking persons, with bony deformities are the people who will benefit from CF.

4. CHAPTER FOUR

The reaction stimulators and detoxifiers

The three Sulphuris'

CALCAREA SULPH, NATRUM SULPH AND KALI SULPH

(CS NS KS)

UNDERSTANDING SULPHUR

Sulphur the element is another vital trace element and plays a major role of an antioxidant in the human body. It is a part of amino acids like methionine, homocysteine, cystein, and taurine, which have effects of antioxidants against free radicals which are harmful to health. Sulphur also has a detoxifying effect, protecting against heavy metal and transition metal ion toxicity by enzyme inhibition thus preventing their accumulation in the body.

So we can relate this role to the symptom to 'lack of reaction' where an ion imbalance maybe corrected by the sulphur containing cell salts. Let us see how.

CALCAREA SULPH:

1. Purulent discharges, that are chronic and wounds or ulcers that do not heal, but continue to ooze, a yellowish thick discharge that is usually non offensive. This lack of the ability of the body to resolve a lingering infection or inflammatory process is the pathology of Calcarea sulph.

2. Problems like chronic obstructive pulmonary disease (COPD) where cough persists for years together, with expectoration of whitish yellow phlegm, finds great relief with Calcarea sulph. We find that lung function can be stabilised and even improved to some extent when the symptoms match.

3. Another character of Calcarea sulph that I have very often verified is-'ailments from appreciation not received'. They become morbidly ill when they feel that they have done so much but have not been appreciated.

Let me share a case here of Idiopathic Granulomatous Mastitis (IGM)

CASE OF IGM-

Granulomatous mastitis is a rare chronic inflammatory condition of the breast tissue involving formation of inflammatory granulations around the lobules and ducts of the breast tissue, forming one or more breast lumps, congestion, pain, abscesses and fistulae. Although rare, it has been observed in increasing numbers of women during their late 20s and early 30s. The diagnosis can be done by biopsy, as it can rule out malignancy, sarcoidosis and infections like tuberculosis and fungal infections.

A lady aged 35 years, came to me with multiple painful lumps in her left breast. It all started when her first baby was about 8 months old. She had a heavy feeling in the left breast, and felt a lump. She thought it was due to irregular menstrual cycles and ignored it for some time. However, it grew in size and felt like a ball. She saw her gynaecologist and had a biopsy, mammography and ultrasound. It turned out to be noncancerous, and as the breast was warm to touch, it was thought to be an abscess. She was given antibiotics and pain killers which did not resolve the problem. She was then advised to undergo aspiration and a small incision was made. The wound was kept open for drainage, and again antibiotics were given. In ten days a newly formed 'pus balloon' appeared which was again aspirated. I noticed that all through the case taking, her tone was that of lamenting . 'I gave up my career to look after the baby and home, and now no one realises what a big sacrifice I made. I am taken for granted, and not valued.'

We have 'Lamenting, wailing, appreciated because she is not' with Calc sulph very prominent. On 20/6/2014 my first prescription was Calcarea Sulph

200X. Calc Sulph also relates to obstinate suppurations that refuse to heal.

The wound stopped oozing and began to heal with healthy granulation.

Her follow up 2 months later: 'I can feel positive changes happening in my breast tissue. Also I get pus sites, but they are small in size and after rupture, a very small amount of pus drains out. A month later she again had a lump 1 inch in diameter with pain, and Calcarea sulph 200X one dose was repeated. This drained and healed up in a week.

22/12/15: No lumps ever since. All the breast tissue is normal.

Granulomatous mastitis is a chronic and very debilitating condition which is refractory to all other treatment options. It resolved brilliantly with homeopathic treatment.

Here Calcarea sulph 200X has been given as a constitutional dose. Calcarea sulph 30X was given as an acute prescription to help the new collections of pus, which drained out with one dose of 2 tablets.

More of my cases of IGM have been published in the Indian Journal for Research in Homoeopathy- IJRH Volume 16 (2022) Iss.1 cited here:

Potdar S. Effectiveness of homoeopathy for the treatment and management of idiopathic granulomatous mastitis in women: A case series. Indian J Res Homoeopathy 2022;16(1). doi: 10.53945/2320-7094.1063

To summarise the prominent characters of Calcarea sulph-

1. Odourless purulent chronic secretions

2. Non healing wounds, after pus has found a vent. To help healthy granulation.

3. Thick yellow crusts on scalp with chronic oozing.

4. Chronic inflammatory processes going on for years. Ringworm miasm. (Ref: Soul Of Remedies-Rajan Sankaran)

5. Gets used to his complaints. 'Doctor, don't worry. I'm used to this'.

6. Cough/cold/bronchorrhoea/COPD.

7. Affections with thick lumpy secretions that are odourless.

8. Grumbling-His value is not understood by others.

9. Lamenting, appreciated because he is not.

10. Hatred of persons who do not agree with him.

NATRUM SULPH (NS)

Natrum sulph is a princely remedy to start a case of head Injury. Give it in the 50M or CM potency. It will help reduce the cerebral oedema that is fatal in such situations. Even mental effects and long continued ailments that started since head injuries.

I had a case of autism in a child, who developed symptoms after she had a fall from her mother's arms. Natrum sulph 200X as the first dose, began to show marked improvement in the child, very quickly.

Natrum sulph has a tendency to water retention, and NS is worse in humid weather. Asthma, headache, skin diseases and many ailments appear or are worse then.

I have found it brilliant in diarrhoea in humid weather. I once had a little child 1 year old passing loose stools laden with worms, and not responding to the indicated medicine. I retook the case but this time considering the humid weather-involuntary stools.

I chose the 12X potency because the diarrhoea had been there for more than a week, it was severe and resistant, but did not call for a 200X. I wanted something between 6X and 200X and 12X was just perfect for the child.

One dose of Natrum sulph 12X ended the misery. The 'single dose miracle' again!

Some characteristic features of this amazing cell salt are-

1. Asthma in damp weather

2. Frequent urination

3. Obstinate fevers in damp weather.

4. Thin offensive yellow purulent discharges.

5. Sudden morning diarrhoea.

6. Itching when undressing.

7. Dreams of insulted being, delusion-need great efforts to be appreciated.

8. Suicidal depression with impulsive tendencies.

9. Hydrogenoid constitution

10. Gonorrhoeal traits

11. Recurrent or chronic genitourinary tract infections

12. Congenital blepharitis, chronic blepharitis.

13. In urinary calculus, with CP, MP, Sil, FP, NM.

KALI SULPH (KS)

It is the fourth remedy after the trio of inflammation Ferrum phos, Calc phos and Kali mur.

Cough with profuse secretions that are yellowish green. This is its area of specialty of KS and that has helped me in all patients who have a tendency to produce that kind of phlegm.

Kali sulph has its skin affinity with profuse desquamation. Hence in eczema, psoriasis, Kali sulph will improve the condition.

Some prominent indicators of Kali sulph are-

1. Burning, heat, greenish discharges.

2. Better outdoors-feel suffocated indoors.

3. Psoriasis – scaling, exfoliation, epithelioma, cancer.

4. Shifting pains, shifting complaints.

5. Eruptions with thick yellow secretions.

6. Otitis media, mastoiditis, ozeana.

7. Hair falls in patches.

8. Lack of reaction

9. Used as an intercurrent/constitutional/in acute upper and lower respiratory infections with FP CP KM 30X.

5. CHAPTER FIVE

NOTE ON BIOCHEMICS IN URINARY CAL-
CULUS

A typical supportive role of Biochemics in this common, troublesome and recurring condition i.e. renal
calculus can be explained like this-

1. Calcarea phos helps correct calcium metabolism to
maintain solutes in liquid form in urine.

2. Mag phos helps release ureteric spam that holds on
to the calculus, thus helping it to pass out in urine.

3. Ferrum phos helps reduce inflammation inside the
ureter aiding the calculus to pass.

4. Natrum mur has an affinity for the urinary tract,
and the tendency for the formation of calculi. It helps
correct the solute and solvent state balance, to prevent formation, and to help fragmentation of calculi.

5. Natrum sulph helps correct the tendency to formation of renal calculi, and thus to expel the calculus by
fragmentation.

Each of the above symptoms have been verified numerous times, and have led to brilliant cures.

6. CHAPTER SIX

BIOCHEMIC CASES

I am sharing here TWO cases that could not have improved without the wisdom of the Biochemics:

CASE 1

A Case of Ulcerative Colitis:

On 4/8/2015 a 7 years old girl suffering from blood in stool, in recurrent episodes, came with her father. She had been given conservative allopathy treatment, with antibiotics, but bleeding episodes continued. Colonoscopy and biopsy were done, and she was diagnosed as a self-limiting colitis. She was treated in hospital for 10 days with antibiotics, as she had blood in stools for 7 days.

Then six months went well, and again she had blood in stool. Now a colonoscopy was done, to reveal lesser number of ulcers, and was now diagnosed as IBD, (Inflammatory Bowel Disease). She was put on a corticosteroid for three months. Blood in the stools stopped. But when the steroid dose was reduced to 5 mg again she had blood in stools.

The third colonoscopy was now done to reveal diffuse ulcerative colitis. She was now put on another steroid preparation. Three months later steroid was stopped, but the child lost appetite. Also now, any minor infection led to bleeding again. She had to leave school since a year and a half.

She had been given Homeopathic treatment on three different occasions from three different Homeopaths and every time, she landed in an aggravation! So this was the fourth and last time they wanted to try Homeopathy!!

Evolution -

The patient is the second child. Her mother did not want a second child, as there were a lot of differences with in-laws. (Unwanted pregnancy). Her mother was very resentful and used statements like-'Why don't I die? Why don't you die?' She still does not speak to her sister since seven years, as she felt offended by her behaviour. Uses abusive words (but cares for this girl child).The child's mother was very upset with her own mother as she did not help during her pregnancy. She was on bed rest with this pregnancy as the baby descended prematurely. Her husband came home very late at night from work, and he then cooked for her. They had dinner at midnight. Generally she was very poorly fed during pregnancy. (Malnourished foetus)

The Child-

She grins when she enters the room and when looked at. Eyes have a clear blue sclera. She speaks in Hindi, though all at home speak Marathi. She is too sensitive. No one can say anything to her, or even suggest doing something differently; her face changes to fear, cries, withdraws and gets blood in stool. Can't bear any discord around her. Can't bear to make a mistake, becomes nervous. She is a perfectionist. She said, "I get confused whether to play or sleep. I feel weak, (expression-of helplessness, wailing tone)". She expresses extreme fear, and is bewildered.

She can't accept her mistake, can't be told that she has made a mistake. Becomes nervous, weeps and is inconsolable. Will sulk until spoken very kindly too and diverted to something she likes. She says, 'I don't feel good. What can I do if Mamma gets angry? I close the door and cry. She says very nasty things to Papa'.

Dreams-Fearful. Sees a ghost who comes to take her away. Then she can't go back to sleep. She has a habit of looking in the mirror and doing hand gestures, she speaks to her image there. "I like doing hand gestures" says she. She makes her own story world, loves playing alone.

She will only do as she wishes, but has a specific routine. She can't bear to be bathed. Her skin is too sensitive to touch. She says, "I feel very ticklish". She is very headstrong, and rigid. She will not take any suggestion, and becomes nervous.

She eats only specific food, prepared in a specific way, everyday. Vegetable paratha, and cooked lentils. She loves chicken. But can't eat it, as she has an aggravation of colitis from it. She is very anxious about her symptoms and health, and says, "I feel very scared". Her facial expression shows great fear and she speaks in a wailing tone. If there is any argument in the family, she gets nervous and has a relapse.

Rubric: Discords aggravate.

She never has any pain or discomfort in the abdomen. The current status is that she has no blood and has regular stools, since she is on steroids. The parents and doctor are hoping to wean her off the steroid. But when the dose is reduced, she has a relapse.

The child has tried Homeopathy before, but she immediately had a relapse and had to be admitted for blood in stools that was continued for a week. Few months later they changed the Homeopath, but again the same thing repeated, twice.

These are the important features of her case-

Oversensitive 4+

Headstrong

Offended easily, weeps

Perfectionist

Change aversion to

Discords aggravate 4+

Bleeding tendency

Fear, nervousness 4+

Anxious about health

Dreams-Ghosts will take her away

Gestures makes with self-talk

Chicken Desires

Bathing aversion to

This is a highly oversensitive child with an idiocyncratic response that easily gets out of control. Such patients may have aggravation with the indicated remedy. Their system is oversensitive to the similimum. And that is why she landed in an aggravation every time with the Homeopathic treatment!

So before the similimum I started FP CP KM KP 6X, 1 tablet of each, once a day to help her susceptibility more capable to handle the indicated remedy.

A month later–

She is more energetic, happier (Sense of wellbeing)

I continued the same for 1 more month. A month later-less touchy. Chats with herself and moves her hands and fingers (makes gestures).

Few months went well. There were arguments at home between parents. She had a relapse. Pasty grumous blood in stools, sticky mucus and no faecal matter.

Given – FP KM 12x, 5 tablets dissolved in 150 ml water, 10 ml every hour. This time she did not need hospital admission, and recovered quickly.

Over the next whole year, there was occasional blood streaking in stool, from minor causes, which was better with one or two doses of FP 6X.

She tried to re-join school. But she became very nervous when the teacher scolded, anyone. Very anxious about school. Since she has a lot of absenteeism, she is unable to cope with her studies. Feels inferior and not at par with others. Can't sleep. Gets dreams of a ghost who comes to take her. And she again had a relapse.

I was thinking around the remedies-SIL, Calc, Ign, Carc.

But in Reference works, I found-'dreams-a monster, a ghost took me away from my home, to a land of ice'. (Massimo's cases-Sea remedies)

And the only remedy is - Corralium Rubrum.

The Materia Medica reveals-

Corrallium Rubrum- very fragile, too touchy, makes a fuss, believes has to follow a certain regime- otherwise will be a disaster. Haemorrhagic tendency.

Corralium Rubrum 30C was given 4 hourly, along with FP CP KM KP 6x, for 1 week. The episode subsided in a week. After a month, I gave her, her constitutional dose of Carcinocin 200, and Sac lac for a month. But her appetite was still poor. Energy levels not very good. Though mentally she was much less touchy. There still were occasional streaks of blood in stools.

I continued FP CP KM KP 6X, 1 tab a day, for 6 months.

The next year saw her transform completely. She is now bold, takes the phone, answers the doorbell. Doesn't bother if scolded. Takes a bath! She joined a school and could give her exams well. She is now a completely normal child, happy, playful, smart and a bit cheeky as well.

This case is an excellent example of how the patient sometimes needs to be brought to a better level of susceptibility in order that she may be able to respond to the indicated remedy, and not get aggravated by it! I believe that without the Biochemics this child would not have been able to live a normal life.

CASE 2

SPINAL ASPERGILLOSIS

A lady, 31 years old, married and a mother of a two year old child, was referred for homeopathic treatment by a neurosurgeon, on 25/8/2012 for a fungal infection in her spinal cord, not responding to Allopathic treatment.

The two types of fungi that are commonly involved in nosocomial (hospital acquired) aspergillosis, are-

1. Aspergillous fumigatus, and

2. Aspergillous flavus, which is more common in respiratory tract infections.

Both release alfatoxin which is hepatocarcinogenic.

Evolution of the case-

She had gone for an eye checkup and found that she had completely lost eyesight in her left eye. On CT scan it was found that she had a pituitary gland tumour. The tumour was operated on, but she developed meningitis. She underwent lumbar puncture ten times over a period of six months, in an effort to diagnose and treat the infection of these meningeal linings on the brain, and spinal cord. She had taken numerous cycles of antibiotics and now, the CT scan and lumbar puncture showed that she had 'spinal aspergillosis', an infection with the fungus 'Aspergillus Fumigatus'.

This is an opportunist infection developed due to prolonged use of antibiotics, and could be hospital acquired. There were multiple lesions between the vertebrae D12 and L1. She was on steroids and anti-fungal drugs. Steroids, because the inflammatory process causes exudations that can compress the spinal cord. She spent about six months at the hospital for all these procedures.

Presenting symptoms-

1. She had severe low back pain, like a spasmodic, but continuous pain, worse lying on back, worse movement, almost continuous, little relief on bathing with lukewarm water.

2. Low grade fever, ranging from 99^{0}F to 101^{0}F daily every evening since about 2 weeks.

3. Very exhausted.

4. Urticaria with hives appearing on various parts of her body, with itching during the fever.

5. She was better by cold applications.

6. She was constipated, no urge for stool. Stools hard and difficult.

7. Hair loss,

8. Blue ecchymoses on her skin, due to the steroids.

9. She has become 'very sensitive'. Cries easily, and her symptoms worsen when she starts to think.

10. She has weight loss and can't eat when she thinks.

I noticed that she was speaking with a mask face with almost no expressions, even as she said she cries for everything!

Let's take the two striking symptoms in the case-

Face; VACANT expression- Tub, Lycps, Kali-br, Camph, etc.

Fever heat; RECURRENT - Tub, Nat-m, Kali s, Eps-b, Carc, etc.

The first dose was - Tuberculinum 1M, single dose, because recurrent fever, exhaustion and a chronic destructive, inflammatory process calls for it.

Followed the next day by a single dose of Hypericum 1M, as it relates to problems due to injury to nerves. And in her case, it was surgical injury of the spinal cord. Biochemics FP KM CP MP KP 6X one tablet each daily was continued.

A week later she said, her fever was gone, and backache reduced greatly. She felt her energy getting better. I followed her up closely, seeing her every other week. One day she complained of numbness in her limbs. She walked with a wobble. The CT scan shows compression of the spinal cord due to the exudations of the healing process. As there is no natural exit to these, decompression with one more lumbar puncture had to be done. She recovered well from this.

The healing of fungal infection left scar tissue on the cord, compromising its function. This meant difficulty in walking. Her knees buckled when she tried to stand.

She now complained of burning in the dorsal region,

Feeling of exhaustion on slightest exertion, < mental exertion

Weight not improving.

The striking symptoms when repertorised-

back; DEGENERATION, spinal cord- Pic-ac, Naja, Zinc, Phos, etc.

PAIN; burning, smarting; dorsal region- Pic-ac, Naja, Zinc, Sil, etc.

mind; MENTAL exertion; agg- **Pic-ac**, Naja, Zinc, **Phos, Sil** etc.

EMACIATION; mental exertion agg- Pic -ac, Ars.

I now gave her Picric acid 200 1 dose a day, for a week. This medicine relates to degeneration of the spinal cord, neurasthenia, and resulting muscular debility. I also advised physiotherapy.

A week later she could walk a few steps. The lost sensations in her limbs started improving. Every week she improved steadily. The Biochemic medicines in the 6X potency given were- FP KM CP KP MP 6X.

Let's see why-

FP and KM indicated in the primary and secondary inflammatory processes,

CP as the primary cell salt relating to aiding cellular metabolic healing processes,

KP and MP - the nerve healers,

All of which working in a fine coordination helped her spinal cord to recover faster.

Can nervous tissue heal?

Neural progenitor or stem cells have been found to exist in the adult Central Nervous System, which are capable of migration over very long distances, and extensive axonal arborisation even synapse formation. This then implies that nervous tissue can heal to some extent!

The outcome-

She showed me her progress sometimes in person, sometimes by video sharing, and how she started her two step walk, then walked from one room to another. She progressed to climbing up stairs, then down the stairs, and then walked with a walker in the garden, then without a walker. Eight months later she came to see me in person, a haversack on her back, walking independently, her face beaming with joy and gratitude. A magnificent recovery with Homeopathy with the knowledge of Biochemics!

7. CHAPTER SEVEN

QUICK TIPS —

1. Deworming - CP NP 12X, 2 tablets each as one dose.

2. Diabetes- CP KP NP NS 6X, OD or 12 X weekly.

3. Cholesterol -CP KM SIL 6X —1 tablet OD

4. Hypertension – FP CP NM KP 6X solution –in 150 ml, 10 ml 2 hourly.

5. Thrombolytic- FP KM CP CF SIL 6X , 1 tablet OD.

6. Cold cough - FP CP KM 30X + KS 30X, (if productive and yellow/greenish) 5 tablets in 150 ml water, 10 ml 2 hourly.

7. Fever- FP CP KM 6X 10 tablets each in 150 ml water, 10 ml 2 hourly.

8. Severe spasmodic cough- FP KM CP MP KP 30X, 5 tablets in 150 ml water, 10 ml 2 hourly.

9. Asthma - FP CP KM MP NS 30X, 5 tablets in 150 ml water, 10 ml 2 hourly.

10. Gastro enteritis FP CP KM NM KP 6X, 5 tablets in 150 ml water, 10 ml 2 hourly.

11. Urinary calculi – to fragment and expel CP MP NM NS 6X, 1 tablet OD.

12. Renal support- FP CP KM KP NM NS 6X, 1 tablet OD.

13. Osteoporosis - CP SIL CF 6 X, 1 tablet OD or 12 X weekly.

14. Wound healing- FP KM 6X locally

You will now easily be able to figure out the reasons for each cell salt in the combinations if you relate them to the underlying pathology.

8. CHAPTER EIGHT

NOTE ON POTENCY

In conclusion, the potency question has always been tricky. But generally, the 6X is to be used when there is more tissue irritation. The 30X when the subjective symptoms are more vibrant, like the patient is more animated to express them. I would use the 12X as an intercurrent. It has an action between the 30X and 200X in terms of the depth and duration of action. So weekly doses as required by the patient. The 200X would be a constitutional prescription. Use in a single dose and do not repeat till its action is exhausted.

There are some highly susceptible individuals who do well even with a single dose of 6X. So the sensitivity of the patient will finally determine the potency and repetition. The same way as applies to any other Homeopathic medicine.

SUMMARY

If we try to understand the 'why' behind the symptoms of our Biochemics, we are led to the study of ion functions in our body, opening up a whole new understanding of the interconnectedness of the cellular ions, and the striking correlation with the symptoms of the Biochemics. Thus multiplying the possibilities of using them wisely for enhanced treatment outcomes.

It is always helpful to have an attitude of a researcher, to prove and verify with keen observation, all the principles and laws of our science, with an unprejudiced mind to explore their scope, limitations, and possibilities.

REFERENCES

1. Boerricke W, Dewey WA. Twelve Tissue Remedies of Schussler. 3rd ed. Philadelphia, PA: Boerricke & Tafel; 1893.

2. Boericke W. Pocket Manual of Homeopathic Materia Medica. 9th Ed. New Delhi: B. Jain; 1991.

3. Phatak SR. Materia Medica of Homoeopathic Medicines. 2nd Ed. New Delhi: B. Jain Regular; 2016.

4. Mitra BN. Tissue Remedies. B Jain Pub Pvt Limited; 2005.

5. Hahnemann, Samuel, et al. Organon of Homoeopathic Medicine. 19 June 2019.

6. Rajan Sankaran. The soul of remedies. Bombay, India: Homoeopathic Medical Publishers; 1997.

7. Mac Repertory Ver 8.5.X and Reference Works Ver. 4.5.2017.

8. Nimni ME, Han B, Cordoba F. Are we getting enough sulfur in our diet? Nutrition & Metabolism [Internet]. 2007 [cited 2019 Oct 28];4(1):24. Avail-

able from: https://www.ncbi.nlm.nih.gov/pmc/articles/PMC2198910/

9. Weiner, Charles, et al. Harrison's Principles of Internal Medicine Self-Assessment and Board Review, 19th Edition and Harrison's Manual of Medicine 19th Edition (EBook) VAL PAK. McGraw Hill Professional, 18 Nov. 2017.

10. https://www.researchgate.net/publication/345311542_A_Solution_for_the_-Heart_a_brief_biography_of_Professor_Sydney_Ringer_MD_FRS_1835-1910

12. Indian Journal of Research in Homoeopathy Vol 16 (2022) Iss.1

ABOUT THE AUTHOR

Dr. Swapna Potdar graduated from D.S. Homeopathic Medical College in Pune, India in 1996, before completing her D.Hom (UK) an Advanced Diploma in Classical Homeopathy from The School of Homeopathy Devon UK in 2009. She then completed her MD in Homeopathy from the Maharashtra University of Health Sciences in 2011. She has always been an ardent student of Homeopathy, and a favourite speaker frequently invited for seminars, symposiums, and continued medical education forums to speak on various topics, especially Biochemics. She is a mentor to students, and Homeopaths from different countries. Her practice though based in Pune, India, spans all continents for over two and a half decades. She has published papers based upon her clinical experiences, in International journals, and her work is freely accessible on the internet. Her research paper published in the Indian Journal Of Research in Homoeopathy (IJRH) on the Effectiveness of homoeopathy for the treatment and management of idiopathic granulomatous mastitis in women, Vol 16, Iss.1 2022 describing a case series of eleven cases is the first of its kind in Homeopathy in the medical condition.

'Hpathy' the popular online Homeopathy Journal recognized her work by awarding her the 'Award for excellence in Homeopathy' in 2022 for her contribution to the field of Homeopathy, on the occasion of the 20th anniversary of the Journal.

Besides her medical practice, she is an amateur artist, pianist and poet. Her book of poems, 'Whispering Petals' has received the Emily Dickinson award.